THROUGH THE SCARS

RISING from CANCER

PASHA CHANEY

Through the Scars: Rising from Cancer

Copyright © 2020 by Pasha Chaney

ABOUT THE AUTHOR

Pasha Chaney is an artist, author, and creative entrepreneur. Having journaled her own cancer experience, she realized she could help others who are experiencing similar life-changing events. Pasha wrote *Through the Scars: Rising from Cancer* as a way to offer others faith, hope, and inspiration. As a cancer survivor and champion for those walking the path of recovery, Pasha gives advice from her heart.

DEDICATION

This book is dedicated to all the newly, past, and recovering cancer patients all over the world, no matter your age, race, color, or creed. May you rise up from feeling hopeless and helpless to feeling loved, inspired, and whole! After reading this book, I hope you feel capable, strong, and resilient to face all of your challenges on this journey of a lifetime, but not the one you expected.

I am also dedicating this book to all the loving caregivers and family members who provide love and support to cancer patients. May you also feel celebrated and confident as you walk through this test with your loved one.

Lastly, to my cousin, Alicia Williams (my birthday twin), I miss you dearly. You fought a good fight, and may your soul continue to rest in love.

~Pasha~

Contents

FOREWORD

"You have INI-1 deficient sinonasal carcinoma." I delivered that statement with gravity to a young vibrant woman in the prime of her life. Most people are familiar with breast cancer, lung cancer, prostate cancer...something that is publicized, we may hear about a breast cancer run or support group for prostate cancer, but not many know about cancers of the head and neck. Head and neck cancer patients suffer silently. Head and neck cancer is devastating to a patient, most of our senses allowing us to interface with the world are through the head and neck allowing us to enjoy many of life's pleasures. This includes our face which for most is their identity. We take life sustaining breaths of air through the head and neck, taste the richness of food through the head and neck, see the beauty of the world through the head and neck, we kiss a loved one using our head and neck and the list goes on and on.

Head and neck cancer treatment frequently consists of a combination of surgery, radiation, and chemotherapy which is both physically and psychologically challenging and even when the treatment is done survivors must deal with lingering repercussions. With many other cancers, the scars are all internal or can be hidden under clothes. When we take someone's taste for food, ability to speak, or in Pasha's case the gift of sight, and we ask them to carry on living happily because they are cancer free, it isn't so simple. They can't taste the food at the restaurant, people have trouble understanding you and keep conversations short at the party, you are bombarded with blank stares with them wondering "why is that person missing an eye?" They carry the scars of their treatment both physical and internal as daily reminders of what they went through. As a cancer doctor with access to state of the art technologies, it is humbling to see no matter how advanced our treatments are, there unfortunately is always collateral damage. We try our very best to minimize it, but we are not trained on how to put someone's life that has been uprooted by cancer into some sort of normalcy. We try to help keep those scars hidden but it's our patients that learn on their own to rise above them.

It never ceases to amaze me seeing how resilient cancer survivors are when they are able to push through and thrive. They are my heroes and are a daily reminder of how resilient humans can be. Here is a story of an amazing beautiful young woman in her prime, full of independence raising her young daughter, blindsided with my words when we first met. Losing one's eye, then going through radiation therapy and chemotherapy is devastating enough. On top of that it is happening during the COVID pandemic where there is so much uncertainty in the world, it's enough stress to put anyone into severe depression. Not Pasha Chaney...she gets through her surgery, is going through chemotherapy and radiation therapy, caring for her young six year old daughter including making sure she is getting her schoolwork done remotely, and tells me she is writing a book. Let me be clear, Pasha is writing this book while still going through chemotherapy and radiation therapy. Talk about true inspiration, when your world turns upside down and you decide you are going to make the world a better place by sharing your story. It is my distinct honor to introduce a true hero in every sense: Pasha Chaney.

Samir H. Patel, MD
Consultant, Department of Radiation Oncology
Associate Professor, Mayo Clinic College of Medicine and Science

INTRODUCTION

*Rise: an upward movement,
an instance of becoming higher.*

Thursday, January 16, 2020 is the day that changed my life. That was the day I was diagnosed with what I thought was summer, seasonal allergies that turned out to be cancer. It turned my world inside out. I never once imagined having cancer in my 30's. No way, no how could I have imagined my life would take such a dramatic turn. But it did and here I am, fully immersed in an experience that has transformed my entire outlook on life, health, family and friendships.

According to the CDC (Centers for Disease Control), 1.6 million people in the United States are diagnosed with cancer each year (CDC, 2020). We all either know someone who has cancer or have personally been affected by it.

Before I was diagnosed, I was a relatively healthy individual. To be honest, I was rarely sick and only had a cold maybe once a year; and I cannot remember the last time I had the flu. I've never had a broken bone, a sprained ankle or anything significant growing up as a child; no major surgeries or emergencies that impacted my life on a daily basis.

However, in a matter of months, that all changed. What started as a very subtle eye watering, nasal drip and frequent headaches turned out to be a tumor the size of a walnut inside my left nasal cavity throughout my left eye socket. My cancer symptoms started growing more intense over the course of time.

Take my advice: Don't ever wait or hesitate to see your doctor for any reason. If you don't get anything from the words I write, I hope you walk away with a sense of urgency when things feel wrong. Time is so critical when a medical condition like a tumor is discovered. If it weren't for a routine eye appointment with the optometrist, I would have wasted critical time before discovering my malignant mass. Once my optometrist sent me to an ophthalmologist, I knew there was a serious problem. I thought that maybe I had a thyroid issue because my eye would not stop watering and was beginning to protrude outward. I tried to diagnose myself with something minor that I could compartmentalize as an "inconvenience" in my life. At the time, I didn't need another inconvenience. As a single mom raising an autistic child, working a full time job and pursuing a creative career in music on the side, there was no room for even an innocent trip to the eye doctor. My life was already hectic, stressful, burdensome, tiring, exhausting, and hard with long days and lots of sleepless nights. Just the idea that I could be sick and not be able to give 100 percent to my daughter and all the things that spread me so very thin was scary and debilitating. However, in all actuality, it turned out to be my "saving grace." My diagnosis allowed me to slow down, even prior to the global pandemic that has put America "on hold."

I had a sort of premonition that everything about my physical self was worn down; my intuition was telling me that something was seriously wrong and out of whack with my body. My legs were weak and pained. My hair started to shed. My body was fatigued and achy all the time. I was running on fumes. The thought in my mind was cancer. It was like I kept being drawn to the word CANCER like a magnet and those who have or had cancer that I've known over the years kept running through my head. Every time I would drive by a building, the words, "Cancer Institute' or "Cancer Clinic," would appear, or I would hear a commercial or advertisement regarding cancer. It was like someone was reading my mind or sending me a message. That's when my thoughts were so strong, and I could no longer ignore the signals I was getting all around me. As it turned out, my premonition had, unfortunately, become my reality.

On March 3, 2020, less than two months after being diagnosed, I underwent surgery to remove my cancerous tumor, which resulted in an enucleation of my left eye, a deep 10 inch scar on my left leg to replace a vein in my face where my eye was removed in order to allow blood circulation to flow properly through my face on the left side, and a skin flap between the base of my skull and frontal sinuses as a barrier to help stop the spread of the cancer to my brain.

I know a lot of this is medical jargon but trust me, when the complicated procedure was explained to me by all my specialists, I was completely overwhelmed and unprepared for what was to come and how my looks and appearance would change. I was also totally unprepared for how I would feel emotionally after undergoing such a major procedure.

I cannot tell you how afraid I was. I cried often; most times by myself. In the beginning, all of the fear and tears had me blinded with the thought that there was no light at the end of the tunnel. But I want you to know that there is a light at the end of every tunnel, and a victory to be won after every battle. I am living proof.

Some days I felt like I was walking through hell, but every day I lived to rise another day. That's what this book is about. Rising through the scars of cancer, the physical and emotional scars of a journey that at times feels like walking through the depths of hell. But scars heal and there is life to live after diagnosis.

My hope is that you will find this book to be uplifting and inspiring. As you walk with me through my journey, you will see how important resilience and vigilance is in the face of adversity.

Pasha Chaney
risingfromcancersurvivor@gmail.com

CHAPTER 1

Rising from the Unknown

Into the Unknown

I came across a meme on Instagram that said, *None of this was on my vision board but the way my faith is set up I will adjust.* I actually made this my life motto after my cancer diagnosis. My mom used to say, "Pasha, life is a series of adjustments and change." As a kid I never liked change or the unknown. I would cling to everything and cry when I lost anything (gloves, shoes, hats, boyfriends, and so much more). Like most people, I love stability, familiarity, and predictability. Life seems to just flow easier that way; at least it does in my mind. Not only is cancer a very scary thing but being diagnosed right before a global pandemic makes this whole experience even crazier.

Facing two unknowns, having cancer and entering into a pandemic is something that left me numb, without words, and debilitated to the point of defeat, before I had time to understand what I was up against. Not only did the global pandemic of 2020 change the world and how we interact and interface with others socially, it also changed the way patients receive treatment. I remember that moment during my mask simulation for radiation... how petrified I was laying on that cold, metal table with a mask as thick as a brick placed over my face. Just me, without my family because the pandemic changed the rules. I had to go it alone. There was no one to hold my hand in those moments or tell me everything was going to be okay. No visitors or family were allowed on the Mayo Clinic campus where I was receiving treatment. Every entrance had a checkpoint with staff taking temperatures and asking screening questions about Covid-19. A high temperature would automatically disqualify you for treatment until you were cleared, and Covid-19 tests were mandatory every 30 days during treatment at the Mayo Clinic. Mayo had very stringent, but necessary, restrictions and requirements to keep everyone safe. However, it wreaked havoc on me as a new cancer patient. I think the shear process of being alone during my mask simulation, chemo injections, and a myriad of weekly medical tests made me feel very vulnerable and helpless during the pandemic. There were so many unknown factors and variables about my cancer, and the information regarding the corona virus seemed to be ever-changing as far as how a person could contract it, and the precautions the entire nation needed to take... until further notice.

Some of my appointments were scheduled as telemedicine visits. Telemedicine appointments are video call visits with a physician. Unlike being in the office, the physician calls you to discuss your medical needs and questions. All of this was new and foreign to the providers as well as the patients. It definitely made the patient-to-doctor relationship a little more awkward, especially during the pandemic.

I didn't like it that I had to talk to my doctors and some members of my care team over the phone, but I'm glad it was available at the time so it wouldn't disrupt my treatment. I couldn't afford to let my diagnosis and treatment schedule be delayed. I needed surgery and treatment for my cancer, and I needed it ASAP! My team of doctors worked quickly in the pandemic to ensure I had the proper tests to determine if my cancer had spread throughout the rest of my body. I was relieved to know that they were using every tool they could to ensure proper timing of my treatment plan. I really can't brag enough about the wonderful staff at Mayo Clinic in Phoenix, Arizona. They are all so kind, respectful, compassionate, and determined to see me through my journey. I needed that in the worst way.

If you have kids I can bet that you have probably watched the Disney movie, "Frozen 2," a gazillion times. As a side note I think the first Frozen was better than the second film (just my opinion don't mind me, LOL). Anyway, what stood out to me the most was the song in the "Frozen 2" movie titled, "Into the Unknown." The first time I heard the song it was highly annoying. High pitched and just the right amount of word repetitiveness to make a parent go crazy! It's unbearable when it gets stuck among the chatter in your head at the weirdest times. But the thing that stands out the most to me about the song is Elsa's willingness to go into something totally foreign and unknown to find herself and who she was ultimately, while celebrating this awakening. As she repeats, "Into the unknown" over and over again, I realized it is a celebration of fully immersing yourself into what scares you and what you fear. That is what cancer is like when you are in the midst of it. If you fully immerse yourself and embrace the challenge and not view it as a daunting defeat, you can come out VICTORIOUS!

During this unknown period, this is the type of chatter that raced through my head, day and night:

- What if my cancer is terminal?

- How long will I live?

- Who will take care of my daughter?

- What if I'm not able to work?

- What if I have to move back home with my parents or get a full-time caregiver?

I even thought about all the milestones in life that I hadn't accomplished like getting married, having more children, and fulfilling some of my lifelong passions. I want to reach my destiny. Everything that I ever wanted to do suddenly became urgent on my bucket list. Have you ever felt like your life was just one big scrambled puzzle and as soon as you start to figure it out, something knocks you down, totally unexpected and out of the blue? Well that's how I felt about cancer. Like it arrived on my doorstep as an unwanted, uninvited, and unknown guest with a look of anger and disgust.

An unknown guest is never wanted at your house. As kids we used to say, "Let the doorknob hit you where the good Lawd split you!" In other words - be gone and goodbye! I wanted to say goodbye to cancer just as fast as it came into my life, but the reality was I needed more than just an "old saying" to ward off this demon. I needed to look this unknown guest straight in the eye and say, "I didn't invite you in, but I'm sure going to walk you out!"

Being Diagnosed

Once your medical physician diagnoses your cancer after multiple CT, MRI and PET scans, including a complete a biopsy, you finally come to terms with the fact that your cancer is indeed real. You have to acquire a mentality to go into fight mode if you want to live and overcome this disease. The mental fight is just as important as the physical fight. I know being diagnosed with cancer may feel like the end of the road, but it isn't. It's typical to have various feelings surrounding cancer and sometimes all those feelings hit you at once. Feelings of sadness, depression, loneliness and isolation are all common, including feelings of anxiety, worry and stress, which we will talk more about in depth later. The truth is, cancer doesn't spare your feelings. It doesn't care about your feelings. It doesn't care about what you had planned next week, next month or even next year. It comes as a disruption, the loudest disruption you never want to hear. It's a distraction that's unwanted to say the least. But if you focus on taking care of your mental and physical well-being in the midst of your diagnosis, you will have the tools to fight a good fight and not let cancer overtake you.

Learning All About Your Type of Cancer, Diagnosis and Treatment

I was diagnosed with nasal carcinoma, one of the rarest

cancers in the United States. Only 2000 people a year are diagnosed with squamous cell carcinoma in the nasal cavity; that's less than one percent of the population (ASCO, 2020). I can't tell you how many times I played the tape over and over in my head on how I could have possibly developed this disease. I never worked in carpentry or a sawmill or anything of that nature. Nor have I ever smoked a day in my life, so it was quite bizarre (actually shocking) to learn I had nasal cancer.

Once I had the diagnosis and status, I wanted to know and learn all about squamous cell carcinoma. I found that the most informative and educational websites were those from the Mayo Clinic. Currently, there are only three Mayo locations in the world (Rochester, Minnesota, Jacksonville, Florida and Phoenix, Arizona). The Mayo Clinic is best known for its extensive and expansive research in disease detection, prevention, and treatment.

I was blessed and fortunate enough to receive treatment at the Phoenix, Arizona location and was referred by a friend who received treatment at Mayo after going through throat cancer three times. Her story was miraculous in itself and provided me hope and encouragement, which I will talk about later.

After speaking with the physicians at Mayo, I wanted to know the best treatment for my type of cancer. Of course, I'd heard about the standard radiation and chemotherapy used to treat cancer patients over the years, but I wanted to know all about the new and innovative treatment for cancer patients in the 21st century and all the great strides the medical professionals made within the realm of cancer treatment.

Proton therapy was recommended by my radiation oncologist and medical team. Proton therapy is radiation that uses a high energy beam to treat tumors and target specific tumor areas. Think of your tumor like a rock. With "regular" radiation the rock/tumor is spray-painted with the treatment. You tend to have more areas exposed and affected outside of the tumor area which can cause damage to other parts of the body. With proton therapy you are "painting" the rock (aka tumor) directly, which protects other areas around the tumor, especially vital organs and sensitive areas. Proton therapy is used to treat certain cancers and is not radioactive so you're able to be around your family once your treatment appointment is complete. The cost of proton therapy is higher than standard radiation.

Proton therapy also has side effects which include fatigue, dry mouth, headaches, possible hair loss, and redness around the treated area.

It is important for you to understand your treatment plan and approach. Whether you decide to complete traditional treatment, modern treatment, or try a holistic approach, you need to be 100 percent comfortable with your choice, and so should your family. You also need to be ready for the anticipated results.

I was also recommended a platinum chemotherapy called Cisplatin. I cannot lie, the thought of chemotherapy scared me. I had heard all the horror stories about patients who take chemotherapy and their body changes. Most people who are not familiar with the different types of chemotherapy have seen stories of patients who lose significant weight on chemotherapy drugs.

Concerned about physical changes, like hair and weight loss, mouth sores, inability to eat, nausea and vomiting was my number one concern. I also had numerous questions about possible infections while taking chemotherapy and how my immune system would be compromised. I didn't want to look and feel sickly while fighting this horrible disease.

I was prescribed Cisplatin and it seemed to work well for me. I was able to maintain a healthy weight, keep food down, and resume some of my daily living activities like work and self-care management.

Telling Your Family

It's important when you're first diagnosed to have all the facts regarding your cancer before telling your family. Of course, they are going to have a lot of questions that you probably can't answer, but there will be plenty that you will be able to talk about. Lots of people know about cancer but are not familiar with the process of diagnosis and all the countless appointments and tests that come along with it. I don't suggest telling your family about your diagnosis over the phone or through a text message, unless you live out of state and have a plan to communicate thoroughly about the information your physician(s) is disseminating.

Once you've shed all your tears, did some self-reflecting and processing, you are ready to tell your family. Everyone will have a different reaction, so you must be ready for it. I really don't suggest you do this before you have had the chance to learn more about your type of cancer and the treatment you are considering. You must be the level-headed person in the room, even though you are the patient.

It's key to first share your news with your immediate family circle before telling extended family, unless they are going to be a part of your caregiving team. I suggest cascading the information in phases to your family. There are reasons for this. One, first you must get the urgent news to your very close kin. These are your foundational family members like your parents and siblings who will likely be your daily support system while you go through this experience. You are going to need their support as much as possible, both physically and emotionally, to help stay grounded and feel loved during this entire process. Then communicate your diagnosis to additional family members and friends who you may not talk to every day but will definitely be concerned about your well-being and want to give thoughtful words of encouragement along the way. Trust me, you're going to need both of these support systems when facing, fighting, and standing up to cancer.

Telling Your Child(ren)

If you have children, you want to ensure their feelings and emotions are taken into account when they learn about your disease. Don't keep them in the dark, no matter what age they are. If you are a parent with a small child like me, it is important that you explain your diagnosis in an age-appropriate way so they can understand. Because my daughter was six years old at the time of my diagnosis, I didn't feel the need to explain the complex process of cancer and how cancer cells invade the body. Instead I focused more on the fact that I had a tumor and that the tumor had invaded my body and I needed to have it removed. I also explained to her that I would need surgery and someone to help assist us at home after the surgery. Lastly, I explained to her that my appearance would change, and I would look different after surgery. I briefly explained the eye enucleation process as well and that I needed to have my left eye removed to prevent the tumor from spreading to other parts of my body.

Just like your family, your child is going to have a lot of questions about your cancer. It's okay to show your vulnerability during these moments, but also provide some security and assurance that you are going to do everything you can to answer their questions. This is all so new. You have no idea how your children will react. Even in your own moments of despair, you must be strong for them.

The goal here is to make your children part of your journey without making them feel isolated while it is going on. In the beginning, my daughter had a lot of questions like,

Why are you sick?

Why do they need to remove your eye?

What happened to your eye?

When will you feel better and we can go back to the way it was?

You must understand that kids have worry and anxiety about your sickness as well. Try to put their mind at ease by carving out some time to talk to them when they are showing signs of concern. I also got into the habit of randomly talking to my daughter about my diagnosis just to periodically gauge how her feelings may have changed or what her interpretation of things were. Asking questions like,

Do you have any new questions about my treatment?

How do you feel about my new appearance?

Are you feeling scared or concerned about me?

I found that once I started to engage more in conversation with my child about everything that was going on with me, it seemed to ease her fears and calm her spirit. We all know kids are like sponges. Not only do they absorb language, but they also absorb and pick up on our feelings and emotions, both positive and negative. Although you may not feel your best every day on this journey, please keep in mind that someone is looking up to you daily and thinks the world of you, and that your strength is amazing. Most likely that person is your child. Even if you have adult children, they are rooting for you and hoping you pull through with flying colors. They are your biggest champions. When you hurt, they hurt; but when YOU win, THEY win! If you have children, assure them that you're up for the task and will give it everything you've got to beat this thing and get back to a life that is whole, healthy and joyful. Tell them how much you love them.

CHAPTER 2

Rising from Negative Thoughts

Thinking the Worst

I'm not going to sugarcoat this at all. When you're first diagnosed you think the worst. The first thing you're probably going to think about when you hear the news is if you're going to die. Well, the truth is one day you will die but that doesn't mean you'll die from cancer.

In 2018 according the American Cancer Society, cancer deaths declined nearly 26% in the last decade (cancer.org, 2020). These declines are in large part to less people smoking and early detection and treatment.

I bet you thought I was going to quote all the cancer deaths in the United States each year. Well no, I actually want to use reverse psychology here and talk about dispelling all the negative thoughts you have about cancer.

Is cancer serious and nothing to play with? Of course, it is, but does it have to be the very end of your tunnel? No, it doesn't. Do people survive from cancer? Absolutely, YES!

If you go into this journey with a negative mindset and stance it's going to affect your overall health and the way your body responds and reacts to stress, which can further complicate your disease.

Rewind to January 16, 2020 when I first learned I had cancer. I mentioned earlier that my body was stressed and strained to capacity. In my opinion, DNA cell changes, a weakened immune system, along with chronic stress were also contributing factors to my health woes. There are mixed reviews in the medical field about stress causing inflammation that leads to greater cancer risk, but one thing I do know is that when you are physically under constant stress you are not well-equipped to fight off foreign invaders in your body.

I began a downward spiral of negative thoughts right before I got sick. Let me be clear. I have always been a positive person who spoke positive affirmations and sentiments over my life, but my mindset started to turn negative because I was mentally and physically tired.

I was a single mom of one raising an autistic child and had never been married. I felt somewhat trapped in my life with constant stress and anxiety while taking care of my special needs child. I'm not sure if you know this, but the amount of stress a special needs parent has is insurmountable.

The emotional strain of caring for an autistic child and worrying about the well-being and care is 24 hours a day, 7 days a week. There is no break. My everyday life was in constant "go mode" with very little rest to replenish my days. In no way am I blaming my child for my medical condition, but I do realize that the amount of stress caring for my daughter day in and day out put me at risk for being overloaded and burnt out.

According to the (CDC) Centers for Disease Control (2020), one in 59 children are diagnosed with an autism spectrum disorder. Autism affects the nervous system and causes difficulty with communication and interaction.

I didn't know much about autism growing up and it wasn't highly prevalent back in the 80's when I was a child. Even now the subject is still very complex and has a wide range of indications when it comes to where children are on the "spectrum" (condition that is not limited and can vary). But now there is more information out there for parents and caregivers including support groups and organizations for parents to utilize. Organizations like "Autism Speaks" www.autismspeaks.org and "Autism Society" autism-society.org are great tools for learning more about autism.

I have a special love for children, especially special needs kids. Before I had my daughter I worked as a Program

Manager at a residential facility for kids with all kinds of needs. We called them "milleus." The job was intense. Some kids were expressive or had very little verbalization skills. Every day was different. Some days were peaceful and calm; other days were chaotic and hectic. You never knew when a child was going to have a "crisis," but you always had to be prepared for any and everything.

I can recall a day I worked on the milleu and I had to de-escalate a child for several hours after a meltdown with the help of my staff. Those some real challenging and grueling days! Learning all about autistic kids and their "triggers" was something new to me back then and also rewarding after taking the time to understand them and their needs.

I would go on to have many more of these types of experiences working with children as a Program Manager. Each day I went into work with the sheer will and determination to help one child at a time. I never backed down from any challenge on the milleu, no matter how tough it was. I looked at that job as an assignment from God and treated it with the utmost level of integrity and delicacy. That's how I view my own daughter - as a special assignment from God to oversee, protect, guide and teach so that she can live a life filled with hope, tenacity and a bright future.

To begin with, it's extremely important that ALL parents, especially parents of special need children, take care of their own physical health. In my case, I wasn't eating healthy and in hindsight, I think my body had very little protein and nutrients to ward off my cancer, even though I was always the one who never got sick. I barely had time to eat so I ate quick foods, snacks, and fast food. I knew junk foods and fast foods were bad for my body, but my lifestyle was totally off track when it came to eating healthy food. I wanted to cook more, but I just didn't have the time. My days would start off like this:

5:00 a.m. – Wake up time and shower

6:00 a.m. – Wake up my daughter, get her dressed and fix breakfast

7:00 a.m. – Out the door for morning school drop off

8:00 a.m. – Morning commute to work

9:00 a.m. to 5:00 p.m. – Work

5:00 to 6:00 p.m. – Evening commute

6:30 p.m. – Pick up daughter from after school care

6:30 p.m. to 7:00 p.m. – After school care commute to home

7:00 p.m. to 8:00 p.m. – Homework, dinner, bath and bed

These 15 hour days, 75 hour work weeks went on 5 days a week, and by the weekend I was exhausted and only had time to sleep enough to have the energy to do it all again on Monday.

After working all these hours, I noticed I started to not care about much, except for surviving on a daily basis and not living and just really enjoying life. That's a dangerous phase to be in, especially when it comes to your health and well-being. I was at a point where I didn't care about anything outside of my daughter and work. I accepted my fate in life as a worn out, tired mom going through the rat race of life while never getting ahead. I could not see the light at the end of the tunnel. It was a long, long tunnel.

I'm saying all that to say this. If you've gotten into a negative mindset and thoughts about your life and how hectic it is, STOP yourself immediately and do something about it! It's not going to do you an ounce of any good by having a negative outlook, unless you want to change it. What you need to focus on is asking yourself:

What can I do about the life I have and make the necessary changes to live a better life when all of this is over?

1. *Am I going to work harder or smarter?*

2. *How am I going to change my lifestyle and reduce my stress?*

3. *Do I need to seek a new job with less hours?*

4. *What things in my life are priority versus what is irrelevant?*

5. *What am I going to put in my body to replenish myself daily?*

Once you start to break those things down you can simplify your life and start eliminating some of the high risk factors that possibly contribute to cancer. Your 'new norm' after cancer is going to require you to dismantle all the negative thoughts in your head with more positive and loving ones; and trust me, **it can be done if you're committed to changing your thought patterns.**

Why Did This Happen to Me?

I don't care what you say, you're going to ask the cursed question, "Why did this happen to me?" That's what I asked myself. Cancer is such a daunting thing and we've all heard the saying, "Why do bad things happen to good people?" We see it happen all the time and question why it happens to us and the people we love. Well the truth of the matter is, all things happen to all people. We ultimately do not control everything that happens to us. The only thing we can control is how we respond to it. I know that sounds cliché, but it really is the truth.

I couldn't understand why I would get sick in what I thought was about to be the prime of my life. I was really looking forward to being financially and professionally established in my career. My personal life wasn't quite where I wanted it, but that was my next goal after settling into my career. But here is the thing. Cancer is no respecter of person. It doesn't care about your age, your color, creed or origin. It doesn't care about your future plans or what you had going on prior to your diagnosis. To be honest, this is the most grappling concept to accept. Cancer interrupted my life.

At first you're probably going to feel sorry for yourself and that's okay...momentarily. But you can't stay in that self-pity forever. Don't get stuck there. If you stay in the "Why did this happen to me" phase, you will be crippled. You have to pick yourself up, dust yourself off, and "Try Again" (which will forever be my favorite Aaliyah song). You can't allow defeat to set in. We all know people who have the 'woe is me' attitude, but in all honesty, has it ever helped their plight in life? NO. There is no sense in having a pity party about cancer. The only party you need to have is the one when the physicians tell you your cancer is in remission or that God says you are totally healed with no signs, symptoms or trace of the disease!

Anger and Disappointment

Some people get angry at God when they get sick or receive a terminal illness, but the truth is because we live in a fallen world, sickness and disease will always be a part of this Earth. I don't believe God wants us to be sick. He wants us to live a whole life to the end of our appointed days. Mind you I said, "appointed" days. So that means sickness and diseases try to creep in to shorten our appointed days. But we can't let this world rob us of a fulfilling life we were meant to live. Then there are those who get disappointed when they've received the status of cancer.

I was one of those people.

I thought, "Why would I get cancer of all things?!"

I'm out here just trying to live a peaceful, prosperous life and take care of my daughter. I never killed, robbed, or cheated anyone. There are so many people in the world who do these types of things and seem to go unpunished. I started to associate good and bad deeds with having cancer. Actually, I tried to justify in my mind who should have bad things happen to them and who shouldn't. I know that may sound crazy, but your mind can take you to so many thoughts when you try and rationalize why you have cancer. But you can't rationalize it. You can only deal with it. It's not a mystery that you have to solve and defend why it happened to you. You only need to prepare for the task at hand and that task is focusing more on the reality than the anger.

Lastly, feelings of disappointment will probably settle in during some point in this journey. Disappointment about how you got to this point in your life, what it all means, what is the purpose of your existence, and how you feel you may have not met up to your life's expectations.

I think I started to feel disappointed through my cancer journey right after my surgery. It was a window between diagnosis and treatment. I really didn't feel like myself. Not only did I look different, I felt different as well. It's like I shed the "old me" involuntarily. I wasn't ready to let the old me go. It happened so abruptly that I didn't get a chance to fully process all my feelings of disappointment that were intertwined with anguish. I felt let down. I felt I let myself and others down. The expectations I had for my life was slowly slipping away into an ocean of regret. But the funny thing about regret is, we only regret what we don't do and for me cancer wasn't a matter of do or don't do. It was a matter of life and death and wanting to live, no matter how my life looked afterward, both physically and emotionally.

Feeling Abandoned and Walking Alone

Feeling abandoned and alone is one of the common feelings to have with cancer. Although most of us know someone who has been affected by cancer, not all of us know someone who is currently "living and breathing" cancer on a daily basis. For a cancer patient, there aren't always many people to talk to right in the midst of treatment or recovery who can relate to what you are going through.

So many times, I felt alone and unable to express my thoughts about cancer. None of my immediate friends had it and no one in my age group had it that I could swap and share stories with. I definitely felt alone and isolated. Although I have people who I know care deeply for me, it just wasn't the same as talking to someone who had my sickness and my type of disease.

Cancer is very rare in younger patients and children. According to the American Childhood Cancer Organization (2020), one in 285 children are diagnosed with cancer, which is estimated to be about 15,780 children a year between the age of 0 to 19.

There are only 80,000 cases of cancer in young adults between the age of 20 to 29 which make up 4% of the population in the United States, according to the "American Cancer Society."

Walking into the Mayo Clinic for daily treatments, I can vividly remember being one of the youngest patients there. I even shied away from saying my birthdate too loud as I approached the check-in counter. I was a minority among a minority population of cancer patients being in my 30's as a newly diagnosed person, so it was very critical for me to seek out additional support.

I can't express enough how important it is to find resources and outlets that tailor to your age population and treatment needs during your journey. It is the difference between walking alone and walking through the fire with an incredible amount resilience and like-minded partners.

No One Understands My Pain

I think 'walking alone' and 'no one understands my pain' kind of goes hand in hand. As much as people try to empathize and sympathize with a cancer patient, they don't fully know how it is and how you feel about cancer unless they have walked in your shoes. That's just the reality of it. You can tell a person all day long what it's like to be living with cancer, but I don't think anyone who hasn't walked this path would truly understand.

In the beginning, I tried to seek out anyone I could think of who had cancer and was around my age, but that list kept coming up short. I couldn't really think of anyone but older people that I knew had gone through it. All of them were 50 and older and had been married, divorced, or had grown children. I couldn't recall anyone who had a small child at home like I did with similar challenges I had like still maintaining my job, a mother with a young child and single. It wasn't until I started talking about my situation through conversation that the dots began to connect for me and who I could relate to.

You'd be surprised who is willing to help and support you once you vocalize your condition. For me, it was a private email from a coworker once I told my teammates at my job about my cancer. A co-worker reached out to me to say that she had throat cancer three times several years ago. I couldn't believe it! I saw her a few times and she was always so bubbly and outgoing. Never once did I think she had ever battled cancer. She was able to tell me her story and how her cancer was in remission. She pointed me in the direction of the Mayo Clinic after she went for a second opinion from previous doctors and was dissatisfied. Her mother had also survived cancer and she shared her mom's story of recovery and remission. My co-worker became an angel to me as she walked me through questions to ask my physicians and oncology team. She also offered me great advice on how to manage side effects of treatment like nausea, fatigue, sun burn and rash from radiation, plus she prayed for me, sent me faith scriptures, and constant, encouraging texts weekly just to keep my spirits lifted.

Not only did I have one angel, but I had two. In addition to my newly-formed bond and friendship with my co-worker, an additional co-worker stayed with me periodically the first three weeks of my diagnosis until my family was able to arrive from out of state. This was a scary time, as I was concerned about living in a city with no immediate family. She was extremely compassionate toward me, as her mom previously had cancer and ensured I made it to my biopsy surgery appointment and rested at home while I was in recovery. She even helped me transport my daughter to school in the morning to eliminate me driving and exerting too much energy. By the time I had my biopsy surgery and found out I had cancer, I was running very low on vitality. I'm so grateful to both of these women who now call me their sister in faith and stand with me in prayer for my complete restoration and healing.

Lastly, my third angel was also a co-worker. I met her during the new hire orientation, and we have stayed connected throughout the years. She sent me a beautiful, handwritten letter of encouragement, which I hold dear to this day. Friendships like these are cherished tremendously. Sometimes your co-worker can become more like angels than friends in a crisis.

I'm telling you, once you open up to the idea of sharing your story, you will find that many people are willing to give you love, support, and encouragement. Don't be afraid to speak up regarding your cancer and try to locate a person, a group or community of those who share your journey.

Emotions vs. Reality

Emotions are subjective, temporary feelings that are not permanent. Remember this as you are going through your cancer journey. Feelings of sadness, anger, and loneliness will go away once you put things into perspective.

The reality is that cancer can happen to anyone, but you have to be willing to push through emotions that make you feel defeated, conquered, and depleted. **You can only control how you respond to the external events around you and not the actual events themselves**. Once you focus on this, then you can begin to feel more equipped to handle your emotions on what may seem like a roller-coaster of a ride through cancer.

Some days you may feel sad out of nowhere and that's perfectly fine; let it happen, but then be determined to pick yourself up out of such a negative emotion and persevere.

You will have many emotional days with cancer, but you can get through them. I remember waking up one day in April of 2020 a complete emotional wreck. Out the blue I started to feel "closed in" by my cancer. When I say closed in, I mean suffocated by the overwhelming feeling of disparity. This was the kind of disparity that felt like a disconnection from the world. Like my cancer had disconnected me from my own life and everything that I've ever known to be true about who I am. There are many kinds of disparities: health disparities, economic disparities, education disparities, etc., but what I call a feeling of cancer disparity is feeling indifferent to the world and parts of you that you feel you no longer connect to.

On any given day, my emotions with cancer would hit me at the least expected time but I took the stance that no matter what I am going to face each day, I would do so with determination and dedication to see my diagnosis and treatment through. Through my recovery phase, I'm going to be a victor and not a victim. Having this type of attitude can help you live in reality (the present) and not be stuck in temporary emotions.

Emotions come and go. Don't make decisions based off of emotions. Try your best to stay level-headed when going through this journey and edify and uplift yourself daily. Whether that's reading books on cancer surviving patients, articles on the next medicines and treatment for cancer, or having a daily devotion or affirmations. I find it helps tremendously when you feed your spirit positive emotions while facing the reality of cancer.

Reality says we will get through this without letting our emotions take over. The reality is your emotions want to cloud your judgment as a cancer patient. Emotions want to take precedence over your logical thoughts and reasoning, but you need a balance. You don't want to bottle up all your emotions while having cancer, that would be highly unrealistic and very dangerous. It's also unhealthy for your mental and emotional state. You must find a balance with how you are feeling and what needs to be done on any given day. You don't want to "live" in only your emotions and be an overly emotional with cancer. If so, how will you cope, handle stress and have the mental fortitude to fight? You would be drained and depleted. You need to have a healthy release of emotions and a strong sense of reality to help process your thoughts about cancer so that you stay grounded.

CHAPTER 3

Rising from Anxiety

Anxiety About Treatment

You ever been scared of the letter "c"? No, not c in the alphabet, and not just the letter c for cancer. For me, I was scared of the letter c as in "chemotherapy." Lots of cancer patients feel anxiety about treatment. We all have these preconceived notions about chemotherapy and what chemotherapy patients looks like. The male patient with no hair or the female patient with a scarf, a thin posture and bedridden for months and months on end. These are the predominant images we see on the television, in the mainstream media, and in a lot of cancer commercials. Sadly, these are the images that are imprinted in our mind when we think of cancer treatment, and that's when it causes an increase in cancer "anxiety."

I wasn't familiar with all the different types of chemotherapy medications and the type of setting that is required for each individual patient to have chemo administered. Not all chemotherapy patients are bedridden. When I entered treatment at the Mayo Clinic in Phoenix the chemo unit was filled with "pods" that included semi-private, reclining chair booths, rooms with beds, and lounge areas with patients all around. This is far different from what I've seen in the media. This is in no way to discount or discredit the patients who are terminally ill and on extended stays at the hospital, I just was very naïve to every person's different plan of care for chemotherapy.

I can recall a day in May 2020 when I went in for chemotherapy treatment and I was very present in that moment and just observed all the people around me. To the left of me was a woman who had ovarian cancer. I know this because she was talking quite loudly to the nurse. But she was also very outgoing and walking around frequently. Her chemo booth had a partition around it, and she had multiple chemo regiments that day. She was up walking around and talking to various staff on the injection floor. Adjacent from me was a woman who had to wait on her treatment due to her platelets being low. She looked tired, her face was pale, but she was in good spirits. I briefly glanced over at her and she reclined her chair to take a nap while waiting to hear back from her physicians. Directly in front of me was a gentleman who was in and out quickly with a "chemo port" placed in his vein and he was able to leave and immediately resume his daily activities.

Again, I must reiterate that cancer treatment comes in many different forms and methods of administering. Hopefully this will help ease your anxiety regarding chemotherapy treatment.

My anxiety and concern revolved around the fear of becoming too sick to do anything for myself and my child. I didn't want chemo and radiation to totally "knock me off my feet" and leave me helpless to fend for myself. I would say knowing what my treatment options were and the success and side effects of the treatments were my second most concern.

I never slept well before my chemo infusions. Without fail, I would wake up in the middle of the night with anxiety. Sometimes I would be up until 3 or 4 a.m. My stomach would be in knots and my thoughts would be in shambles. Sometimes my body would wake me up just to see if I was alive the next day, that's how bad my anxiety was. Sounds totally cryptic, but it's true. Anxiety at night also caused me to sweat profusely. I was inundated with constant thoughts of worry about how chemo would change my appearance. Not in a vain way because I've never been a vain person. It was in a way that tore apart my identity and the bodily characteristics of my physical imprint.

Before my cancer I loved taking pictures with family and selfies on social media to show my personality to the world. But that all changed. It's no secret that your appearance is connected to your self-esteem and can tie in with your self-worth. When you have anxiety about cancer your self-worth can become diminished. It's important that you still feel good about yourself and your appearance, even while you are going through cancer. Your self-worth isn't determined by Instagram "likes" and "views" or any social media standard for that matter. Wake up every morning and still get dressed, groom yourself, and take care of your hygiene. You may not feel like being in large crowds or around a lot of people when going through cancer treatment but be sure to "show up" for yourself every day. Take pride in how you look, even with the changes within and outside your body. Your body is your temple, take care of it. Pamper yourself if needed and give your body and mind some rest and relaxation time. A little TLC (tender loving care) goes a long way when you have cancer. Fight your anxiety by doing things that give you peace and tranquility.

Anxiety Regarding Caregivers

One of the most important things after diagnosis is knowing who will help take care of you and if you'll need their full-time of part-time support. Most patients turn to their family who they feel the most comfortable with who can take time off work to help during this process. Unfortunately, not all family members can take FMLA (Family, Medical Leave Act) to care for their loved ones. This can put a strain on your loved ones and contribute to determining who will care for you when you're sick.

I was blessed that my mother, who retired five years prior to my diagnosis, was able to assist me during treatment. My mom stayed with me a total of four months - before and after surgery, as well as during chemo and radiation. My sister also came to help relieve my mom so she could get a mental and physical break from driving me to appointments to cooking and cleaning and ensuring my daughter attended all her zoom meetings during distance learning for school during the pandemic. In the midst of treatment, these days were long, hard, and tedious. My family, including my mom, sister, brother, stepfather, cousin, and uncle all rallied around me during my greatest time of need and became a very strong and stable support system for me.

Sadly, after I shared my heartbreaking news about my diagnosis, it seemed to be a ripple effect of sickness in my family. It was like the devil was trying to attack my entire family with sickness and disease. My brother got sick with the flu and was in the hospital, my biological father had a stroke, and my sister wasn't feeling her best.

My heart sank, as I wasn't sure if my mom could handle taking care of my daughter and me physically and emotionally, with both of our needs and challenges. Not only did she have to support me and take me to my numerous doctor appointments, she also had to help me manage my daughter's home school timetable. She had to help me manage all of this while being away from her support system which was my stepdad. They had been married for 32 years and he had come into my life when I was 6 years old. He had always supported my mother and had been a strong presence in our lives as a family man. He flew out to be by my side during surgery. During the time he was back at home, my mom was missing him and missing his support in the process.

Although my stepdad or biological father couldn't physically be my caregivers because of their own health conditions and distance, they both provided the emotional and at times financial support that I needed during my concern about care.

I don't want my mother to take on all the physical burden caring for me and I needed to put into place a plan to have care even after she was gone. I decided to do some research and contact some Home Health Care Services like Comfort Keepers and others to see what my options were. A lot of these companies will come into your home at a reasonable price. Don't be ashamed to receive in-home help. It doesn't mean that you'll need home aid forever. It just means for now you are being smart about how you plan to have assistance with your daily living skills, house cleaning regiments, meal preparation, and cooking. Being comfortable with how you will live in your home before, during, and after treatment is key to your success.

Anxiety Regarding Job Status

Jobs can be so unpredictable. In today's world, most people don't spend 30 plus years at a job and retire anymore. Gone are the days of our parents. Work can especially be uncertain when you run into a medical condition that may put you out of work for a significant amount of time. I had been at my job for five years and still I worried about the reaction of my team and those who I had worked with for years. Of course, your employer can't fire you if you are covered under FMLA (Family Leave and Medical Act) during your condition (that would be considered discrimination). But you do have worry and anxiety about the sustainability of your job during your medical crisis. You will also worry if you will be able to return to work and perform at the same level of adequacy and at the same capacity. There's a long "laundry list" of things to consider when having anxiety about how you're going to put bread and butter on the table.

If you can work during treatment, that's great; and if you can't, that's fine, too. Don't beat yourself up about time off when it comes to your health and wellness. You are the most important person here. Take all the time you need so you can get back to your life the way you need to. If you were to leave this world today, your boss will find a replacement for you; but your soul and individuality cannot be replaced in this world of seven billion of people. If it's going to boil down to your job and your life, please choose the latter.

Medical Bills and Financial Anxiety

Now I know I just told you that if everything boils down to taking care of yourself and your job, take care of yourself. This is absolutely true, but if you do decide to return to work because of financial reasons, I would definitely understand.

After my surgery and treatment, I was thousands of dollars in debt. Although my health insurance did cover a portion, I was still reasonable for the rest. Imagine worrying about medical bills coming in, in the middle of a global pandemic where most of the economy is shut down and going through cancer. That in itself will keep you up at night! You're going to have to find a way to balance your finances and your diagnosis. It's like you have to compartmentalize the two and not think about them simultaneously. When you're at treatment, think only about treatment. Be fully present in that moment. Ask all the questions you need to about your treatment and how your body will respond to medication side effects and how you will feel on an everyday basis. Also, to keep in mind, have a specific time when you sit down to review your incoming bills. Do it on a less stressful day when your mind is clear and you're free from negative thoughts. Perhaps you like to review your bills during your morning coffee or with your breakfast or even when your kid(s) are down for bed or after dinner. Whatever works best for you, just make sure you do it when you have time for yourself. Set up payment plans and make arrangements if you cannot pay your medical bills in full. Don't let your bills stress and worry you. Look at your budget and figure out the amount you can afford to pay without going into debt and having a delinquent account. There are also tons of cancer patient funds that help assist patients with medical bills. Connect with a social worker on your team at your medical institution to find out how you can apply for these funds. Some require you to provide proof of income to be qualified for these funds while others administer a quick questionnaire about your diagnosis and needs.

Anxiety Regarding Body Changes and Appearance

The fact of the matter is that your body is going to change at some point when you have cancer. Whether that's internal or external, there will be signs that your cancer is within you. You may feel fatigued or have hair loss, you may lose significant weight, your nails may become brittle and break easily. You may have mental fog, experience lymphedema (swelling of the arms legs and face) plus changes is sexual function and fertility. Also, you may experience severe pain in the cancer area that may make it hard to get out of bed. All of these things could occur when you have cancer; plus going through cancer treatments will cause your anxiety levels to rise.

For me it was the hair loss and weakened legs that made it unbearable to walk and even stand at times. Including the minor cuts and bruises that didn't heal easily once I had cancer. Cuts, scrapes and scars that would normally take a few days to heal started to take weeks. This was all very new to me and I had lots of apprehension about myself in the mirror and how I looked to others.

I've never been the one to be vain or shallow about looks, but for me it was the sheer idea and concern that I would not be able to present myself in the outgoing, creative and fun manner that I was used to. I loved taking "selfies" on Instagram and posing videos of my life and music. Something I started to immediately shy away from once I learned of my cancer. I started to hide behind my diagnosis, which is something I definitely don't recommend to others. That being said, I do understand the need to uphold your integrity and presentation of yourself to the public during your experience. There should be no rush or push to feel obligated to succumb to the pressure of engaging in social media, social activities, and outdoor engagements to validate who you are. You are more than enough even in your feelings of anxiety. Remember, this anxiety is temporary and will pass over time as you feel more confident about yourself during recovery.

Anxiety About Being Inadequate

Inadequate is feeling less than, unequipped, and incapable. We've all felt this in our lives but as a cancer patient, you feel it 10 times worse. You may feel inadequate to care for yourself, your home, your child(ren), pay your bills, and inadequate to overcome cancer itself. You may also feel your purpose on this Earth doesn't quite add up to what you want or what you thought about your life.

I can recall a time after diagnosis that I didn't feel adequate and up to the task of persevering through what seemed like an impossible mountain to climb. I like to use the analogy of a hiker who prepares for her trail. She chooses her location and maps out her "game plan." Once she decides on her location she figures out the terrain and all the tools and equipment she may need for her journey. She even brings along emergency items in case something unforeseen happens during her trip before embarking on her journey. Well, how do you feel adequate enough and prepare for a journey like cancer? In essence you do the same thing. You learn everything there is to know about your cancer and all the treatments available. Just like the hiker and discovering the terrain, you ask your doctors how long your cancer journey will be. Six weeks of treatment, three months or longer, and what will it look like for you on an everyday basis? Lastly, on your cancer journey, have some things in your "trip arsenal" to prepare you for emergencies. Your faith-based books and materials to keep you going when you feel anxious about what's going on in your life, including a close-knit group of family and friends that you can call on in the darkest of days. If you approach your anxiety this way, it will help you combat your feelings of inadequacy with preparedness.

CHAPTER 4

Rising from Worry

Why Are You Worried?

Why are you worried? You have cancer. What the heck!
That's why you're worried. I would be worried, too. Not
worried in the sense of panic, but worried in the sense of
highly concerned. Worry is that uneasy feeling in the pit of
your stomach or the back of your throat. It comes in like
waves sometimes after subtle thoughts, then it rages like a
roaring wind. My gosh, there are so many things that you
worry about when you have cancer. And most of the time
they all lead back to your very first concerns: Will I survive?
How will this change and impact my life? Will I completely
recover?

In the beginning, you will probably worry a lot and I do
mean a WHOLE lot! Trust me it's just a part of the process

and its human nature to worry about things we cannot control. We tend to worry about things we don't have much knowledge about and the outcome. Although cancer is still very much present in the world, it is still almost a taboo subject and topic in the sense. I don't mean just taboo because people are afraid to talk about the "Big C" (Cancer). I mean taboo in the sense that there is no conventional cure at this time and there are so many forms of cancer and cancer mutation cells that it's a very complex disease.

Although cancer is a disease and doesn't hold the same stigmas as say sexually transmitted diseases, it still holds a stigma of the unknown. How and why do some people get the disease and others don't? Is it due to bad genes or were some people just dealt a bad hand in life and they just have to deal with it?

I almost thought for a second that I was given a bad hand. I was worried that a series of misfortunate events was going to be a pattern in my life. Here I was in my 30's battling cancer out of all things! Right before my cancer I was having financial woes in the last year that stretched me to the max, my personal goals weren't coming together like I hoped, and my autistic child needed more care than what I could handle. I needed supportive services for her so I could give myself some relief at home. I was constantly worried and was in a total frenzy about my life. I was fretting that cancer was just the "icing on the cake" and would be my demise after all that I was going through and everything that I had been through. I worried that cancer would "take me under" in the figurative and literal sense. I didn't realize I was living with a self-defeating attitude. I had adopted a self-destructive mentality around what I perceived to be a bad life.

If you think that you have a bad hand in life and that's your perspective, then your outlook will be negative all the time. But instead of worrying about life not being fair, look at life as a series of wins and losses, good and bad for everyone and not excluding anyone.

How Constant Worry Steals Your Will to Fight

All I can tell you is that worry is a destroyer of hope. It is the complete opposite of faith and you need three basic things; hope, faith and sheer will and determination to overcome cancer. If you worry and not hope, you are already defeated. You need to go into this battle with the mindset that you will conquer this disease and let that be your "mantra" as you go through this tunnel. No matter how long of a tunnel, all tunnels have an end point and a light at the end. ALL life lessons have a silver lining in the cloud. Focus on the silver lining and that light even when you cannot see your way. You can also think of it as a storm. All storms do not last, no matter how violent or damaging

- they will pass and there will be a time to rebuild and embrace the new. Keep this in mind when you are fighting! Never lose hope or give up or give in. Your mind is a powerful weapon and you can *will* your physical body to come into alignment with your thoughts. That is how great the Creator has made us! We are made in His image; therefore, we can speak and manifest our thoughts into reality, but that can work both ways: in a positive or negative direction. The less you stop worrying and speak positively about your cancer and situation, the more you build your hope and faith that you'll make it through.

Wet Pillows and Sleepless Nights

I would cry until my pillowcase was soaked in puddles during my sleepless nights. This is how I dealt with my cancer feelings and emotions at the onset. The tears would just flow, and I would allow them to do so, without hesitation. I believe tears are a form of cleansing and God knows I needed cleansing from the inside out: from worry, from stress, and the pressures of life. It's really amazing the amount of "dirt and residue" our souls pick up during life experiences and circumstances. From the time we are born to the time we leave this world we experience trauma scars in many different forms and fashion. All scars are not physical. I believe all of our souls are in need of a rebirth and a reset.

Think about a scar for a moment. A scar is caused when the thick layer of your skin is damaged. That means it took something traumatic to penetrate the skin in this manner. A scar turns into a scab. That scab is needed to protect the wound as it heals. A scar is also a mark that is left on the body after healing. The process of healing is an amazing thing. This also lets us know that the body is a living organism that can heal and repair itself. Just like the wounds on our skin can heal, so can our bodies heal from cancer. It is not impossible. The body is complex, yet it also yields the key and hidden solution to our sickness and disease.

As I started to think and worry about my own mortality, I thought about all the people I had unresolved issues with, either personally or professionally. I wasn't at peace with this. I began to do some soul searching and "healing." I'm a firm believer that healing doesn't just take place in the physical realm, but also in the soul realm.

I made a list of people I needed to contact and apologize to. If you're reading this book and I have offended you at any point, please accept this book as my open apology. I wouldn't say I had a long list of enemies, but you never know how you may have rubbed someone the wrong way or they felt you overstepped your boundaries with them in your personal relationships.

I just wanted to wipe my slate clean after learning I had cancer. I didn't care if I didn't have the person's phone number, I reached out through social media, DM, texts and emails. At some point we all have to take responsibility for our actions and how we interact and treat people in this life. It doesn't matter if we think we are a good person or not, we all have room to grow and ways to improve ourselves. Try mending your relationships and making them right. I guarantee you'll feel much more free and lighter in your spirit and your anxiety levels will go down. Having strife and conflict in your heart only leads to more pain and anxiety.

When I think of cancer, I think of it mutating bad cells and destroying good cells. But I'm also inclined to believe cancer can creep in through burdensome life deposits and negative life trauma, so the spirit needs healing and transformation. I'm speaking in spiritual terms, as we believers know that everything in life has physical and spiritual components.

In order to "cleanse" my cancer-ridden soul I began to make amends and apologize to those I had caused trauma on and forgive myself for trauma and scars that happened to me over the course of my life that I couldn't control. This process was very insightful and introspective. Once I got rid of the old residue on my soul from the past, my spirit started to feel lighter and free. That's when I was able to stop worrying and felt fully free to fight my cancer and free of heavy weights that conflicted with my soul.

What's Next for Me?

None of us knows what the future holds, but in every stage of life we've asked ourselves, "What's next for me?" Cancer patients worry about the same thing. We are not immune to this question. It's very important for a person experiencing cancer to take a simple yet practical approach. Simply said, the lesson here is to put your best foot forward one day at a time. Neither live in the past or the future, but in the moment. Cherish each second with your family and loved ones. Take none of those moments for granted. Tell the people you love that you love them while we are all here and never miss an opportunity to show love and kindness.

Living in the moment keeps you less worried and anxious about the future. Allow yourself to feel every emotion in the present without judging, belittling, or condemning yourself for cancer. Your cancer story is unique to you and only you. You get to write and rewrite this story as many times as you need to in order to make a difference and impact the lives of others. We don't always have control over how our story ends, but we do have control over how we mold and shape all the little stories in between our lives to have an impactful meaning.

Worried About What My "*New Life*" Will Look Like

Your life is going to change after cancer, there's no doubt about it. You're going to have a "new norm" that you may worry about and compare it to your old life. Don't be afraid! Your life can change, construct, deconstruct, demolish, then rebuild and you need to be open to it. You may decide to do a full overhaul on your life and change your belief system about life and death after your experience. You may decide to totally change your eating habits and become more aware and conscious of what you put in your body. You also may decide to try new things in life you've never done before and take different risks in your career, love life, and personal relationships. Whatever you decide to do, make sure it's a benefit to your overall well-being.

Lots of people that I know have turned vegan (a person who does not eat meat, eggs, dairy, or any products derived from animals) or pescatarian (a person who does not eat meat but eats fish) after cancer as a lifestyle choice.

According to the National Cancer Institute (2020), red meat (beef, pork, and lamb) consumption is associated with an increased risk in colon and rectal cancer.

I'm not suggesting everyone become vegan or pescatarian, but it is something to consider when contemplating lifestyle changes.

Your new life won't look like your old life, but you can make it better and as fantastic as you want! The good thing about your new life is that you don't have to compare it to anything. Instead, it will be a clean slate for you to paint on a new canvas the memories of your life. Allow your anxiety and worry about your new life to subside and just go with the flow and the natural current and process.

Worried About Limitations

After my extensive tumor surgery, I had multiple limitations which I will go into further detail in the last chapter titled, "Rising Through Cancer." All my life, I had been healthy and now I was worried about my new limitations and disability. I was worried because my confidence level was not the same anymore and I worried about how my limitations would affect my quality of life and ability to work and support myself and my family. A limitation can be a challenge and a hard work-around, but there are solutions. Try to be solution-focused during your cancer journey. This will help you face your limitations with a positive focus. For every problem, there is an answer. If you have a physical disability due to your cancer, take your strengths and apply them to your weakened areas. Motivate yourself to be a winner. no matter what mixed bag life throws at you.

I've watched countless stories and documentaries on people who have lost limbs and organs, now living as amputees. Within all these stories I have found that these individuals are extremely resilient, incredibly strong, and tough. It's unbelievable the amount of strength the human soul has that translates into physical fortitude, once put in a position to do so. You'll never know how strong you are until you're faced with a grueling circumstance.

All cancer patients do not have to get organs or limbs amputated; but unfortunately, there are lots that do. There are tons of women who have undergone double mastectomies for breast cancer, men who've had their tongues removed partially due to throat cancer and on and on. Can you imagine the level anxiety within these sub-group of cancer patients? I can't even fathom it, even in the midst of my own circumstances.

So many take their five senses (taste, touch, seeing, smelling, and hearing) for granted, I know I did - especially after losing partial vision, tasting, and smelling after my procedure. I felt scared and burdened about losing my eye alone.

Honestly, I was worried that I couldn't carry this load. But because I had never been through something of this magnitude I really couldn't gauge if I had the stamina to prevail. But little did I know, I did. I was even stronger that I had ever imagined. It's like when I needed the strength to get through this, I had a reservoir of power that came out of nowhere. Actually, I won't say out of nowhere; it had to come from God.

I would say that limitations only mean you have to do things differently; it doesn't mean you cannot do things at all. Again, don't worry about your limitations, focus on your robust ability to be strong! It lies within you and you probably don't even know it is there. Your strength is at the very core of your existence. It makes up your DNA, just like the cells in your body and the characteristics of who you are. It is a part of you in every facet. Limitations remind us that we are all human, but it also reminds us of how incredibly capable we are!

CHAPTER 5

Rising from Loneliness

Feeling Isolated and Lonely During Diagnosis

Loneliness is a by-product of isolation. Loneliness is the state of feeling sad and being alone. It is possible to have tons of people around you and still feel alone. Think of all the famous people who have lots of adoring fans and still feel lonesome. Or even the spoiled kid in school who seems to have all the material things money can buy, but still feels empty. Loneliness has nothing to do with status and all to do with how a person interprets being alone when no one is around.

Plenty of cancer patients have frequent feelings of loneliness. One of the reasons cancer patients feel lonely is because they can't always participate in former activities with family members and friends that they were accustomed to. Sometimes there just isn't enough energy and stamina to maintain activities that they once enjoyed.

Secondly. Some friends and family don't know what to say, how to talk to, encourage or console cancer patients after diagnosis. Perhaps they are uncomfortable with speaking on these delicate matters, but their heart is in the right place and they don't have the right words.

Lastly, others may just shy away and have a hard time coping with the fact that you have cancer and may go into "flight" mode and leave you hanging because seeing you go through cancer is too overwhelming for them.

The global pandemic of 2020 made it even harder for cancer patients to connect socially outside of their household. Friends and loved ones couldn't stop by because of quarantine and socially distancing guidelines. People couldn't embrace their close friends due to safety reasons. The entire Covid-19 virus separated families in a way that we hadn't seen since the Spanish Flu pandemic over 100 years ago.

Sorting Out Your Lonely Feelings

First identify why you feel lonely. As a cancer patient, did you feel lonely prior to diagnosis or after? Did the global pandemic of 2020 attribute to more of your loneliness? When you are with you friends and family do you feel loved and supported or isolated and secluded?

For me, the global pandemic made me feel even more isolated. I had a lot of alone time to ponder on my cancer, which wasn't good. In the past, having friends to come over was a positive distraction and kept my mind off things: company and conversation was a big help. I longed for and missed the days when being social was commonplace and "normal."

I had to fill my idle time of loneliness with other things and get creative. I found myself reading more books, even writing this book and planning for some goals I had for myself after treatment. I remember talking with my aunt (my mom's sister) who reminded me that she defeated breast cancer. She told me some very key things that stuck with me during an in-depth phone conversation about her cancer and her friend's cancer who had passed away. My aunt told me that my journey would be hard, but I would get through it as she did. She also told me that I would be emotional and cry, and I would get through that as well. But one thing she mentioned is that I needed to have something to look forward to when all of this was over. Something I could think about that would keep me going and some plans I had in the future for my daughter and me. This conversation really hit home because at first I felt like I didn't have much to look forward to. But after I started to have a little glimpse of hope, I began thinking about my long-term goals again, and how I would accomplish them once this was all over. I wanted to get a new place (which I did) to give my daughter and me a fresh start. I wanted to get my finances together and get back to my creativity in some capacity that wouldn't interfere or hinder my "new norm." Once I saw this was possible, my loneliness and isolation didn't seem so prevalent. I had other things on my mind and new things to look forward to.

Another nugget of good information that my aunt gave me is that she reminded me about her friend who had breast cancer and took care of herself for many, many years after her diagnosis. Because she had no husband or family as caregivers, she took herself to doctor's appointments and treatment. She was strong and didn't have pity for herself. She was alone but had the willpower to keep going. Although she passed away years later and didn't have much family around, she had my aunt who talked to her every day. She was alone, but not lonely.

Finding Support Groups

I was able to find and attend a virtual head and neck support group during treatment and the 2020 pandemic. Support groups are great because you can hear survivor stories, relate to people who have similar symptoms and side effects as you, and feel comfortable in a setting with people who have experienced the same things as you have. Support groups provide a sense of solace and togetherness and provide a great source of coping with emotional stress and isolation in a safe setting. I highly encourage anyone who has cancer or is a caregiver of a cancer patient to find a support group to cope with these challenges.

You can find resources for support groups by researching online or asking your healthcare provider(s) for more information. Don't be embarrassed to attend a support group, whether it be online or in person. These groups can help you manage your feelings of loneliness and improve your coping mechanisms.

How Sharing Your Story and Giving Back Lifts You Out of Loneliness

The best way to cope with something is to give back in the area you are facing. Not only does it make you feel good inside, but it gives you a mission and purpose through your pain and scars. Some cancer patients in recovery like to volunteer at their local cancer organizations. Others like to do speaking engagements at local and national churches, conferences, and seminars. Whatever you decide to do, do it knowing it will not only help someone else, but it will help you as well.

For those who cannot commit their time, they choose to donate and give monetarily to many cancer-funding projects. These programs help cancer patients tremendously with transportation, food assistance, medical bill assistance, and homecare assistance.

How Counseling and Talk Therapy Helps

There is a lot of stigma attached to therapy especially in Black and Brown communities, but it is much needed. There are so many benefits to counseling, which include sorting out your feelings, gaining coping skills for your life challenges, self-awareness, putting your life into perspective, finding new ways to change your life, and more.

I entered counseling about four weeks after my surgery. I wanted to give myself some time to physically heal after my tumor removal before expressing all that I was feeling to a counselor, so that I could solely focus on my mental wellness.

I think the difference with cancer patients in counseling is that you have so many feelings all at once that come rushing in, and you need a soundboard - a person to listen and help you unpack those feelings.

If your employer has an EAP (Employee Assistance Program) a program to help employees address personal and work related problems utilize it for counseling services. If your employer doesn't an EAP program or you cannot afford counseling search for some affordable alternatives. Some churches and faith based organizations offer counseling to members through their licensed therapists on staff.

There is no time limit on how long you can and should stay in therapy. Stay as long as you need to so that you can work out your challenges during and after cancer treatment. Therapy makes a world of difference when you are pressing through this journey. Embrace it. Utilize it. Use it.

CHAPTER 6

Rising from Depression

Depression is a feeling of persistent sadness for a significant period of time. There are many different types of depression and some of us may have experienced one form or another of it at some point in our lives. Whether it was depression from the loss of a job, the end of a relationship, or the stressors of life. Depression can seem paralyzing.

According to NIMH (National Institute of Mental Health) depression affects nearly 16.2 million people in the United States.

Cancer patients are commonly affected by depression. Hopes, plans, dreams and goals are often deferred for an unspecified amount of time, which can cause a sense of sadness and depression. It's important that cancer patients talk through their feelings of depression with a trusted loved one or professional personnel. Something as simple as giving a nonjudgmental listening ear and being a dear friend can help a depressed patient talk things through. However, it is important that healthy boundaries are established when cancer patients "vent" to loved ones and caregivers, as this can cause undue stress and anxiety in the one who is supporting you.

If a cancer patient is suicidal, please call the National Suicide Prevention Lifeline at 1-800-273-8255 for help.

What Does Depression Look Like with a Cancer Patient (What to Look for)?

Depression can manifest differently in various people; however, there are certain signs and symptoms to look for specifically in cancer patients experiencing depression. These signs include excessive sleeping (or insomnia), significant weight loss or weight gain, repeated conversations of hopelessness, talk of death and suicide. Any one of these signs can be cause for concern. It's important for loved ones and caregivers to point the cancer patient in the right direction for medical and professional help. Continue to support in a positive way by keeping the lines of communication open to know how the patient is feeling and dealing with depression. Staying engaged with the patient will help you gauge his or her emotional and mental state.

How Cancer Affects Your Mental Health

Cancer patients go through a very specific grieving process related to diagnosis. Those stages are denial and isolation, anger, bargaining, depression, and acceptance. They can be in this order or out of sequence.

In the previous chapters we have discussed isolation and now depression, but we haven't really touched on bargaining and acceptance.

Let's discuss the bargaining stage for a second. When I was first diagnosed, I thought that I could reason and bargain with my doctors about the loss of my eye. Although my left eye didn't have cancer in it, it had to be removed because the tumor had totally enveloped my eye socket and could possibly spread, causing more damage and vision loss. I went as far as to get a second opinion and both times the physicians told me there was no way for me to save my eye.

You can imagine how disappointed and let down I felt. I thought I could somehow bargain my way out of the eye enucleation, but I couldn't. I think that was the thing that affected my self-esteem and confidence the most after surgery. This also made me feel depressed right after I learned I had cancer.

After the doctors very adamantly explained to me that my life needed to take precedence over my eye and that saving my eye was secondary, that's when I began to accept everything that had to be done to save my life. Honestly, it has taken me four months after diagnosis to really accept the new changes in my life. I've had to adjust to a lot of things and how I live and maneuver in order to accept this new norm.

The acceptance phase definitely should not be rushed. It took me four months, but it may take you longer or even a year or more to accept your new reality. There is no timetable on how long it should take you to feel better and more confident about the direction in which your life is headed. My advice is to work through your depression phase until you get to the acceptance part of your journey.

Your caregivers will also go through these grief stages as being a supporter of you. It's imperative that their feelings and mental health are also taken into consideration during this time.

Difficulty with Concentration and Attention

Because of the effects of radiation and chemo on the central nervous system, especially to the head, neck and brain area, cancer patients can experience difficulty with concertation and attention. Memory loss and brain fog can also occur.

I experienced brain fog and memory loss as well when my tumor was growing, since my cancer was in my nasal cavity through my eye socket to the lining of my brain. I remember being slightly depressed because I couldn't remember simple things. I couldn't even write music lyrics and remember them as I was accustomed to doing as a creative. I started to forget things easily in the middle of a sentence. To me it was frightening and embarrassing.

To combat memory loss, I started to write things down and plan my day accordingly. This helped me keep myself more organized. Instead of trying to remember music lyrics at once, I would write them down and repeat them over and over until something "clicked" in my brain to recall the words I said repeatedly over and over again. These were some very trying times and I still do have occasional brain fog during recovery, but now I am able to manage it in a more effective way that works for me and not against me.

How Caregivers and Loved One are Affected by Cancer Patient Depression

Because cancer can be such an overwhelming diagnosis, caregivers and loved ones need just as much support as the patient. It's important for caregivers to understand their level of commitment to their loved ones without feeling depleted and exhausted. Caregivers may also experience depression as they witness emotional, mental, and physical changes with the ones they love.

There are numerous support groups for caregivers as well. I encourage all caregivers to find ways to cope with caring for yourself during such a difficult time.

I constantly encouraged my mother and sister to take time for themselves while they were caring for me and my daughter. Things like going to the park and carving out "me" time was extremely beneficial for them. Getting out the house and going to the store for a "pamper" day was also highly recommended. I wanted to make sure my family stayed sane through this process as well. I didn't want them to feel defeated and become depressed in the midst of helping me. These "mental breaks" played a pivotal role in keeping us all safe and healthy.

Chapter 7

Rising from Fear

What Is Your Greatest Fear?

All of our fears are different. It all depends on how we see the world, how we grew up, our personal experiences, and how well we've handled those experiences. Fear basically means being afraid. So, as a cancer patient what is your greatest fear? Your greatest fear is probably being afraid that you will die from cancer. Secondarily, you may feel that if you don't die will the cancer return and thirdly you may feel if you don't die how your life will look after cancer. All of these are valid fears. But there are two types of fears in this world and that is positive and negative fear. Negative fear causes you to not take risks and stifles you. Positive fear will cause you to push past your comfort zone in reach for something better in life. You're going to need lots of "positive fear" versus negative fear as a cancer patient. There is so much fear of the unknown that you will need to thrust yourself into the sea of the unimaginable. Let your fear turn into faith and propel yourself forward.

Facing Your Fears Head On

There's no use in confronting your fears unless you are going to do it head on. I know this from personal experience. Once I was diagnosed with cancer I had no choice but to face it head on with my feet planted firmly on the ground. A lot of people in my generation like to say "10 toes down" which means you yourself are vouching for how strong you are in facing any situation and meeting whatever obstacle. I like to think of myself as this strong as so should you! You're very well capable of facing your fears if you allow it to shape you rather than break you down. Fear is often an illusion and a projection of circumstances that could happen but that doesn't necessarily mean they will happen.

Keep your eyes on the task set before you and not the fear that you are feeling. Allow yourself to mold your fear into triumph.

Using Your Faith and Spiritual Tools to Overcome Fear

My faith and God helped me the most during this trial and tribulation of cancer. Without my spirituality I would have not been able to make it this far. I can't imagine someone facing something of this magnitude without knowing God and His love and presence over you at all times. When you know God, you know yourself and you know you were born for a specific reason and purpose. You were created with a life mission, we all were.

Perhaps your story is similar to mine or you have a completely different cross to bear. Whatever your cross may be, be diligent in carrying it. Some days you may have to lay your cross down and care for yourself. Other days you may carry your cross and help others in the process with similar situations. It's the way you carry the cross and not the weight of the cross that helps you to endure.

My spiritual tools included my church, my bible, my daily devotional prayer, and various faith-based books. I leaned heavily on my church before and after my diagnosis and received much needed prayer in the process. My pastor and his wife prayed for me on numerous occasions at the church, and so did pray partners. These prayers kept me uplifted and encouraged. My church sent me letters, cards, and emails, and stayed connected with me during this difficult time.

My bible was a resource for me for scriptures on faith and healing. I constantly meditated on *Isaiah 53:5:*

"But he was wounded for our transgressions, he was bruised for our iniquities: the chastisement of our peace was upon him; and with his stripes we are healed." (KJV)

Psalms 147:3 "He healeth the broken in heart, and bindeth up their wounds." (KJV)

There are so many scriptures to meditate on, but you get the point. You can Google "scriptures to meditate on" and you will definitely find one that resonates with you, personally.

I'm a strong believer in speaking God's word throughout your lifetime and saying these things out loud to remind you of the power of God's spoken word.

Prayer also became a part of my daily regimen. Just spending some alone time with my thoughts and God is what I needed to feel some peace and calmness through this storm. Some days I would pray and then sit still in silence for God to come into my heart and give me a sense of comfort. Other days I would just mediate on His word and let the scriptures fill my heart with faith and hope.

Whether you chose to mediate or pray is totally up to you, but when you do it, have a spiritual purpose and a way to connect to the Creator.

Lastly, reading faith-based books was also a tool I utilized on this journey. I read books like, "Eat your Way to Life and Health," by Joseph Prince. It really helped to inspire me to live on in a purposed-filled life.

Joseph Prince's book, Eat your Way to Life and Health: Unlock The Power of the Holy Communion, was recommended to me by my father and it was one of THE best books that I had ever listened to on faith and healing. I bought the book in audiobook as a CD to use in the car and in the house. Prince's book takes the approach of healing the body from within, from sickness and disease, and the power and principles of the Holy Communion and how it ties into the scriptures. This book really blessed my soul and my life. As I discussed in Chapter 4: Rising from Worry, I went back to mending relationships and faults with people during my introspection. This book was a huge factor in that process. I rededicated my purpose back to God so that He could use me, and my circumstance, and my story would not be in vain.

I also started receiving communion on a regular basis as a reminder of my rededication and commitment to God. I wanted to be assured that no matter what happened in my life and with cancer, that I know where my soul lies.

Those communion days helped me realign and refocus on my mission here on Earth. It also helped me remember God had already paid the price for my healing and even in a fallen world with sickness and disease, that we can still speak His word and claim the benefits He has spoken to us through His holy word.

Trusting God

One of the most important connections that you must have throughout your journey is your spiritual connection with God. None of my faith through cancer would have been possible if I didn't have a personal relationship and bond with the Lord. I'm not talking about manmade religion, the type that keeps you condemned and keeps you bound. I'm referring to the ability to bond with the master, the one who created you and has the manual for your life through His love. That's a beautiful thing!

When you are in a trusting relationship with God, the peace that you feel is tranquil and it helps you get through those bad and tough days when it's rough and you're having a hard time coping with all of your issues with cancer. Hold steadfast to your relationship with God during these troubled times. Your faith will always be an anchor for you during those rocky storms that disrupt your life. Don't ever give up on Him, because He will never give up on you!

Hope as an Anchor

Hope is a desire that is strengthened through faith. If you anchor your faith in God's love and His word, you can withstand anything. As I said earlier, it's amazing how resilient we are as human beings. Think about it. We experience love, life, loss, change, and adaptation to unforeseen circumstances, yet for the most part we continue to preserve.

Having hope is that perseverance we need on a constant basis. Don't discredit how powerful hope is on your cancer journey. Let's be clear, hope and optimism are not the same. It is easy to get these two things confused. Hope is based on desire; whereas, optimism focuses on a controlled outcome. We cannot control our lives through every action and reaction. However, we can plant seeds of hope to project our lives in specific directions that we choose.

Have you ever seen people become overly optimistic about a certain thing and when it doesn't work out, they are totally crushed and depressed? That's because they have optimism and not hope. Have you run into those who are viewed as *falsely positive*? They ONLY see the positive in everything and are never neutral to anything. They don't know how to problem-solve when things go wrong and have a hard time processing disappointment. Be rooted and grounded in hope and not optimism alone. The two characteristics go together well, and things get done!

CHAPTER 8

Rising from Cancer

My Personal Childhood Story

I can still hear my parents' words echoing in my ears far more often than they uttered them: "Pasha you're so strong and such a hard worker," and then they would say, "If there is anybody we don't have to worry about, it's you!" I guess I grew up being somewhat tough and strong; at least that's the story my scars tell. I was a product of my environment, having been raised in Flint, Michigan, one of the most dangerous and violent cities in America.

Growing up in the 80's, I was no stranger to family violence. The violence directly impacted and permeated throughout the course of my life and sought hard to define me as a young woman. However, during my cancer diagnosis and treatment, I realized it was the adverse effect of family violence that offered me strength, courage, and resilience to fight back.

I realized in that moment, the very catalyst that desperately and negatively tried to define me was the same catalyst that prepared me for this journey.

My childhood fears were derivatives of a painful family memory of the violence I encountered at the age of six. Following my parents' divorce, my mother remarried, and my father maintained his visitation rights. It was the summer of 1986 when the family violence suddenly broke out after a weekend visit with my father.

The use of physical violence was chaotic, and it forever changed my life, as well as all those involved. It was in that moment that I felt a protector and a warrior spirit overtake me, as I instinctively draped my body over my six-month old brother's body to protect him from the sudden and chaotic danger. The altercation itself left me with an unexplainable scar that remains to this day, running deep like the lyrics in Tupac's song, "Pain."

That same year following a family vacation at Disney World, our family would experience yet more violence. Our home was fire bombed, and we lost everything we had. As a child, this tremendous loss left me with a feeling of emptiness, with no personal items to cling to, as everything was smoke damaged. Our family was displaced, living in a hotel room for three months. According to the Resource

Center on Domestic Violence: Child Protection and Custody (2020), 3.3 to 10 million children are exposed to adult domestic violence each year.

As a child, the family violence seemed to never end. I was torn apart by the fact that, at my age, I had no means to protect anyone from the unthinkable physical and mental pain associated with such cruelty.

From the onset of my diagnosis, this childhood pain challenged me to take on that warrior spirit deep within again and fight for not only myself, but for my precious daughter. Losing everything from the home firebombing was devastating. I didn't have a dress or doll that I could play with, out of all of that wreckage; the house was a complete mess. The loss of so many personal things guarded me internally. Losing things is sometimes painful. I attribute my toughness to those days. It hardened me in a way that didn't make me bitter, but it made me different when it came to facing fear. That is, fear cannot hold me or keep me bound. I had been a survivor of many things, including the destruction and confusion of my childhood and youth. I have been fearless for a long time. I am ready to show my strength!

You ever heard the saying, "pain changes people"? Have you ever thought about what that means? It means that someone has changed their mindset, personality, or belief system due to a pain that they experienced. We all encounter many internal changes as we work through our personal pain, and in some cases, it can be a great catalyst for change. If you allow it, it can propel you forward. Pain can be useful in more ways than one. It doesn't all have to be associated with negative thoughts and feelings. Try to think of a time when pain changed you in a positive direction.

I never again wanted to feel that vulnerable and helpless like I did in that moment when I was six years old. Fast forward to today and I still don't like to see myself too vulnerable in any circumstance. I do my BEST to fight and push through my own vulnerabilities. I feel being vulnerable is good in certain situations but being overly vulnerable can be a detriment to your emotional growth, so I chose not to let cancer put me in a state of constant fear.

That is why I focused on not putting cancer before myself. I was still a person who had a whole life to live. I wasn't going to let pain and vulnerability rob me of that, and neither should you. I'm sure you've pushed through many painful experiences and you came out okay, and probably with more resilience than before. If you have, you're already a winner in my eyes, and already well on your way to becoming a conqueror of cancer! Hold yourself in the highest regard and think of yourself as royalty. Royalty that needs to be protected and respected. Don't automatically let cancer come in and disrespect you and your way of life just because it is a disease. Make cancer respect you by standing up to it, fighting back and giving it a black eye! POW!!!

What I learned from my childhood trauma is that those experiences brought scarring, but it also gave me the resilience to be fearless in the face of adversity.

I'm so grateful my parents rose from their challenges within their marriage, which helped me rise from my challenges. Seeing them change over the years after they gave their lives to God gave me hope. This is the same hope that I will carry for the rest of my life!

Create a Vision Board of Survivors

Because I have a survivor's mentality from all the scars that happened to me over the years, I decided to create a vision board of cancer survivors to remind me of all the people I know personally who have recovered from cancer.

This board consisted of my aunt (my mom's sister) who I mentioned earlier in Chapter 5, my mom's mother, who survived breast cancer, and my mom's brother, who survived prostate cancer. It also listed my great-aunt and second cousin, my cousin's best friend, and on and on. I even included celebrities who have survived cancer, like Lance Armstrong, Sheryl Crow, Pam Grier, Christina Applegate, Wanda Sykes, Robert De Niro, and many, many more.

Perhaps you also need a visual reminder of those who have survived, I know I did. It helps to keep things in perspective for you. It also gives hope that if others can survive, SO CAN YOU!

Changing Your Lifestyle and Mindset

It's no doubt that your lifestyle and mindset will change after cancer. There will be a shift in your thought process. Whether that's living better in general, eating healthier, diving into your spirituality, or taking care of your mental wellness. All and any of these things are vital to your successful cancer journey.

It's also important that you have stress management skills after cancer and try to reduce your stress amount by having routines and regular exercise. Some people take up yoga and meditation, while others do home exercise, Zumba, or dance classes. Others may be more interested in sports to stay active like baseball, basketball, tennis, or soccer. Whichever way you decide to be active, choose something that will fit your lifestyle, body, and overall health. It must be something that you get up every morning to think about! Something that makes you want to get out of bed!

Completing Treatment

Completing treatment is one of the final steps in the process of recovery. At the end of your treatment, you may have many questions and concerns for your providers. Write these questions down and ask them at the end of your last few appointments. Good questions to start off with would be:

1. *Can I have a copy of my end of treatment summary which includes diagnosis, prognosis and treatment explanation?*

2. *What is the likelihood of the cancer reoccurring and how often will I need to be monitored and followed after treatment and for how long?*

Also ask for a list of support groups within your area and any additional resources you may need after treatment. Be fully prepared to ask these questions and keep the information handy in a folder you can refer to later.

Road to Recovery

Everyone's road to recovery will vary, but the good news is being on this new road is a gateway to your new life. You can live well after treatment! Your survivorship will depend on how well you adapt and welcome your new changes in life. Volunteering is also a great way to give back and stay connected with other survivors through meaningful activities, support, and partnership.

According to the American Cancer Society, in 2006 the National Institute of Medicine recommended that every cancer patient receive an Individualized Survivorship Service Plan. This plan should be filled out by your doctor after you are released from initial care to help with improving your life.

What Does a Survivor Look and Feel Like?

You may still have the effects of cancer, even after becoming a survivor. Cancer effects may cause early onset of other ailments like heart problems, early menopause, kidney, and bone issues. On the outside you may look fine, but you may not feel 100 percent. You may also still have bouts of fatigue and neuropathy (finger and foot numbness, pain and muscle weakness). These are the characteristics of a survivor. We don't all look the same or feel the same.

I, too, have experienced leg and muscle pain and cancer-causing fatigue that doesn't seem to go away. I definitely operate under the level that I am used to, but I have found "work arounds" for my challenges. Now I try to pace myself better, including my work and not overdo it. I've learned to work smarter, not harder, which used to throw my body off kilter. I've learned that every day is different. I have my good and bad days, but like the gospel song by Paul Jones, *I Won't Complain.*

After your treatment is complete, there are three stages of survivorship: acute, extended, and permanent. Acute survivorship starts at the beginning of diagnosis, extended survivorship starts at the end of your first treatment round, and permanent survivorship is after years of remission. All are very key steps in recovery. Surviving is about living and living is about maintaining a life you can manage throughout the best and rest of your days.

As I write this book, survivorship for me is still an ongoing process and will be for many more years to come. In total, I have seen almost a dozen doctors, surgeons, nurses, and staff involved in my treatment care. I will have to be monitored by my physicians for at least the next five years with three-month checkups the first few years, then twice a year and once a year to make sure my cancer is in remission. The upside of squamous cell carcinoma is that if it doesn't reoccur within five years, then it doesn't come back. I held on to this very powerful piece of information closely as my doctor explained during my pre-operation appointment. He also informed me that there is something called a "high five at five" where cancer patients celebrate their five-year remission of being cancer free! This conversation gave me multiple things to look forward to as a cancer survivor.

In addition to having medical checkups for the next few years, I am also surviving as an organ amputee, due to my eye removal. I may still need additional cosmetic surgery before I am able to have a prosthetic eye (which is also something I am looking forward to as a survivor in the future). I'm grateful that I will have an opportunity to improve and restore my appearance after surgery.

My advice to you is be a survivor with a winning attitude and a grateful heart. Grateful that you are alive and living, and here to make more memories with family and friends.

Why I wrote
Through the Scars: Rising from Cancer

When I learned I had cancer, I was terrified and didn't really have a game plan at first for what I was going to do. I didn't know if my cancer at the time had spread to other parts of my body. Thankfully, it had not spread, and I wasn't looking at prolonged treatment and hospitalization. My cancer was detected in enough time to preserve my life and for that I am forever thankful to God Almighty!

If you are a current cancer patient or survivor, I want you to know that you are not alone. There are tons of great doctors and resources to help you along the way. Do your due diligence and extensive research. Don't be afraid to reach out to people and professionals for help. Never feel hopeless and helpless on your journey.

Once you get over the initial feelings of being diagnosed, come up with a plan on how to manage your life through all the upcoming appointments, treatment and aftercare, including any home care.

Although I have physical scars from cancer like losing one eye, losing my sense of smell and taste, having a 10-inch cut on my thigh and a skin flap below my brain, I rose to the occasion and so can you! I was expected to stay in the hospital after my 22-hour surgery for quite some time after having such a strenuous operation. I left the hospital in a fraction of that time. I willed myself out of that hospital bed, barely able to walk. I used a walker for the first few months of recovery after my surgery, and I can remember the days I could barely pick my head up off the pillow after head and neck surgery. The human will and spirit is a strong force to be reckoned with, I'm telling you!

Key Takeaways

If you don't get anything from this book, I want you to get this:

1. *You are not alone in your cancer journey*

2. *You can survive cancer*

3. *You can rise though cancer despite your physical and emotional scars*

4. *There is support out there for you and your loved ones*

I urge you to utilize all the information and resources I have mentioned in this book to help you on your path: Talk therapy/counseling, the National Suicide Prevention Lifeline (if needed), and cancer patient support groups for survivors and caregivers. Take the time to locate great cancer facilities in your area with a team of doctors who will care about you. Also recognize friends as angels who will come to your aid when needed. All of these support systems will make you feel loved, and that is essential to your ongoing recovery.

The Goal for You, Your Loved Ones, and Caregivers

The goal is to seek help as needed, find support groups in your area, have frequent mental breaks for yourself and your caregivers to recharge and regroup, and love yourself enough to know that with God all things are possible on this journey and He is with you, guiding you, loving you and rooting for you, *and so am I!*

Take one day at a time with cancer because every day will look and feel different. There is no need to rush your recovery but go at a pace that is comfortable for you. Your life will forever be changed by this life event, but you can transform it into something beautiful that gives your life meaning and purpose. You will find your gifts and talents throughout your pain, struggle, and journey. Cultivate those things and make them your passion. For me, it has been writing. Perhaps for you it will be starting that business you always wanted to start before you were diagnosed or taking that trip or vacation that you keep saying you want to do. Maybe it's even proposing to that woman who you want to spend the rest of your life with or telling that guy you really do love him and you're ready to take the next step!

No one knows how long we have on this Earth and life is way too short to have any regrets! Go out there and SMILE! Live Your Best Life. Scream, *I'm Living My Best Life!* like Lil Duval, the comedian, but live it responsibly. Stop stressing about every little detail in your life and just LIVE! Don't just exist to survive, but to enjoy life. We all have a lot to be thankful for, no matter what we're facing. Change your vibe and change your life. Try to keep your life easygoing, with more gratitude than drama and negative feelings. I'm telling you from personal experience that it works, and you'll thank me for it later (you're welcome. lol). Think about the words I am saying. I want you to end your cancer journey on a high note, not a negative one. Let your songs be in your *key of life*, as Stevie Wonder said back in 1976. Be harmonious and beautiful, like a memorable song.

Because I am an artist and musician, I always associate songs with every phase of my life. We all connect music with a feeling or emotion during times when we feel loss, pain, sadness, joy, and happiness. The best song to describe my life at this moment after cancer would have to be, *Through the Storm* by Keith (Wonderboy) Johnson. We can make it through anything, including cancer, and I hope you believe that from deep, deep, deep in your heart. It's time to find out how strong you can be.

I pray that you also rise above your circumstance and that my words will give you hope, peace, serenity, and tranquility during your cancer journey. God blesses you every day!

ACKNOWLEDGMENTS

Thank you to my daughter, Christiauna, who has pushed me beyond measure to be a great mother and a conqueror of all things.

Thank you to my parents, Joe and Jessie, for always supporting me and being parents, I can count on during any adversity.

Thank you to my biological father, Dana, for recommending so many spiritual books to me over the years that sparked my creativity in writing and being an author and artist.

Thank you to my brother and sister, for always having me and Christiauna's back no matter what.

Thank you to my cousin Kai and Uncle Matthew for being by my side during surgery.

To my "special angels" Kenna, Kimberly and Christina: thank you for your friendship and compassion.

To my church family at New Heights in Chandler: thank you for the countless prayers!

To my McMullin, Chaney, Houston, and Ryan family: thank you for covering me by faith with your prayers.

Thank you to Dr. Samir Patel, M.D., Tia Scott, Bianca Houston, Sparkle Harris, and Tyra Hill.

To the Mayo Clinic in Phoenix, Arizona, thank you to the staff for taking such good care of me and making me feel like a patient and not just a number. Because of all of you, I am a survivor!

REFERENCES

ASCO, *Cancer Data and Statistics,* 2020. Retrieved from
https://www.cdc.gov/cancer/dcpc/data/

ASCO, *Childhood Cancer Statistics,* 2020. Retrieved
from https://www.acco.org/childhood-cancer-statistics/

ASCO, *Colorectal Cancer Prevention,* 2020. Retrieved
from https://www.cancer.gov/types/colorectal

Autism Spectrum Disorder: From Numbers to Know-How. (2020). Retrieved from
https://www.cdc.gov/grand-rounds/pp/2014/20140422-autism-spectrum.html

Grief and Bereavement, (2020) Retrieved from
https://www.cancer.org/treatment/end-of-life-care/grief-and-loss/grieving-process.html

Prince, Joseph, (2019) *Eat your Way to Life and Health: Unlock The Power Of The Holy Communion,* Harper
Collins, NY.

Resource Center on Domestic Violence: Child Protection and Custody *Effective Intervention in Domestic Violence and Child Maltreatment Cases: Guidelines for Policy and Practice*, 2020. Retrieved from https://rcdvcpc.org/resources/effective-intervention-in-dv-and-child-maltreatment-cases.html

"*Survivorship Care Plans*," 2020. Retrieved from https://www.cancer.org/treatment/survivorship-during-and-after-treatment/survivorship-care-plans.html

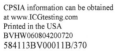